THE CULTURE OF THE ABDOMEN

EXERCISES FOR WOMEN

SEX AND EXERCISE

A STUDY OF THE SEX FUNCTION IN WOMEN AND ITS RELATION TO EXERCISE

By ETTIE A. ROUT

(Mrs. F. A. Hornibrook)

FOREWORD BY

A. C. HADDON, M.A., Sc.D., F.R.S.

DEMY 8vo.   6s. NET

"It is my belief that the health of the womanhood of England would be vastly raised towards the ideal if what you teach could be brought home to the lady who lolls on her Chesterfield as well as to the washerwoman standing at her tub. The human body becomes deformed from overwork just as much as from laziness; and if you, by a miraculous propaganda, could bring home to women, and men too, that most of us could be upright and supple at 55 if such exercises and dances as you teach were practised daily, something would be accomplished you might be proud of."

SIR ARTHUR KEITH, F.R.S., M.D., F.R.C.S., LL.D.

"The importance of the muscles which are attached to the female pelvis has not hitherto received the full measure of attention which it deserves. Amongst the women of the leisured classes, by the wearing of tight corsets and high-heeled shoes, these muscles are encouraged to atrophy from disuse, with the inevitable consequence of the displacement of the pelvic viscera. Dislocation of the bowels causing constipation and all its attendant horrors is one result; displacements of the womb, with their attendant nervous phenomena, is another. These are commonplaces with the medical profession, and if the public fails to heed them it is certainly not for want of hearing them. Miss Ettie Rout's interesting and courageous book advances the subject many steps further. The measures which she advocates are based on sound anatomical and physiological principles, and, if adopted as widely as they deserve to be, they cannot fail to lessen the incidence of disease and to improve the appearance and promote the happiness of women. In any community the health and happiness of the women is the pivot round which the peace and prosperity of the people revolves."

LEONARD WILLIAMS, M.D.

THE CULTURE OF
THE ABDOMEN

THE CURE OF OBESITY
AND CONSTIPATION

BY

F. A. HORNIBROOK

PREFACE BY

SIR WILLIAM ARBUTHNOT LANE, Bart., C.B., M.S.,
Consulting Surgeon to Guy's Hospital, etc.

FOURTH EDITION

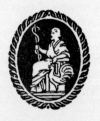

LONDON:

WILLIAM HEINEMANN

(Medical Books) Ltd.

1926

FOREWORD.

I HAVE read the proof sheets of this book with interest. Although it may be true that "there is nothing new under the sun," it frequently happens that we go through life without having seen all that the sun shines upon. When we come across some of these things they strike us as new, or different in some way. The reader will not find any new or startling discoveries bearing on his anatomical structure or physiological functions in the ensuing pages, but he will find described in simple and forceful language a system of exercise original in conception, simple in application, and positive in results. The author's life-long devotion to athletics and all that pertains to physical culture eminently qualifies him to speak with more than an ordinary degree of authority upon such subjects. I feel confident, from what I have seen of his methods, that his claims are not based on mere theory alone.

W. H. HORNIBROOK, F.R.C.S.,
D.P.H. (Irel.).

November, 1923.

LIST OF ILLUSTRATIONS

xi

In lazy Apathy let Stoics boast,
Their Virtue fix'd, 'tis fix'd as in a frost,
Contracted all, retiring to the Breast;
But strength of mind is *Exercise* not *Rest.*"

"Essay on Man."—POPE.

PART ONE

I

INTRODUCTION

I BEGAN active athletics at the age of fifteen. I have rowed as a senior oarsman in Ireland, won prizes at putting the 16-lb. shot and throwing the 56-lb. weight, have done a good deal of mountaineering in New Zealand, Australia and South Africa; have been a long-distance swimmer; obtained the Medallion of the Royal Life-saving Society; have practised wrestling and physical culture, fancy skipping, etc., etc. For over twenty-five years I have practised every known system of physical training, and read widely on the subject. During the war I was with the Australasian forces, and when in the East suffered from sunstroke. I was invalided to hospital in England for three months. My weight on entering hospital was 13 st. 4 lbs.; on leaving 10 st. 12 lbs. Then came 1918 in France, where, though gradually getting better, I was still far from feeling fit. After the armistice I spent several months in Paris, studying hard while there ; and for a year afterwards was in the devastated areas doing Red Cross work. At this time I suffered from a cart accident, and partially paralysed my left arm thereby. This was due to injury of the circumflex nerve of the shoulder. Deprived of the regular exercise to which I had been accustomed for years, I began putting on weight. On returning to England in 1920 I treated my arm myself, with massage and nerve-stretching exercises. To show how completely I recovered the power of my arm muscles, I may mention that I broke the British professional "Crucifix" weight-lifting record on February 9th, 1922, by $11\frac{3}{4}$ lbs., holding $132\frac{3}{4}$ lbs. —viz., 69 lbs. in the right hand and $63\frac{3}{4}$ lbs. in the left hand—the injured arm. I was then forty-three years of age.

Nevertheless, in spite of all this training, and in spite of the fact that I exercised regularly every day, I found myself putting on weight. On July 1st, 1922, I weighed 14 st. $8\frac{1}{2}$ lbs. stripped, which for my height— 5 ft. $8\frac{1}{2}$ in.—was excessive. I then realised I had the fate in front of me of practically all men who go in extensively for athletics : the piling on of adipose tissue in later life. Long walks and diet re-

strictions—in fact, the usual methods employed—
failed to effect any reduction in weight. Although
I looked well, and felt strong, I often found my
work as a masseur exhausting and trying,
especially in the summer-time.

About this time I set myself to designing an
entirely new system of physical exercise. The
system, as perfected by me, is presented in this
book. Briefly, it may be described as a method
whereby it is possible to localise effort to the
abdominal region, to promote more internal
abdominal activity, and to concentrate on correct
posture. Nine months after putting these theories
into practice I weighed 12 st. 9½ lb.—a reduction
of no less than 27 lbs. There was not only a
loss in weight, but an enormous gain in health
and vitality, a greater mental alertness, and much
better functioning of the abdominal organs,
particularly the organs of excretion. Work
which tired me before is now a pleasurable effort,
and the eternal struggle and worry to keep my
weight down is a thing of the past.

I explained my methods privately to medical
practitioners, who were convinced of their sound-
ness, and sent me many patients. The results
have been so gratifying that it has been decided
to publish this book, in the hope that the system
herein explained in detail would be of help to

many people troubled with obesity. But it is equally efficacious for constipation, even obstinate cases benefiting in time.

In writing the book I have endeavoured to omit all superfluous explanations and unnecessary theorising. It may be contended that this book is not a complete treatise on physical training. It is not intended to be. It is not my intention to prescribe exercises for little used and unimportant muscles, or to take in the whole of the four or five hundred voluntary muscles of the body. My object has been to design a system which will cultivate those parts of the body that, owing to man's posture and to his civilised habits, are the most neglected parts of his body, albeit the most important, viz., the muscles of the abdomen and the organs of digestion and excretion. I may add that practical experience shows that the average man and woman soon become tired of ordering their physical lives wisely and well by conscious effort. Therefore, it is of supreme importance to cultivate in them *correct posture*, which in the course of a few months becomes an unconscious habit of body. Correct posture and the occasional retraction of the abdomen during the day (as explained more fully on page 18) will maintain to a great extent the improvement gained by this course of exercise, although naturally it is of very much greater advantage to continue the few minutes exercise required as a daily routine. Considering the supreme importance of the abdominal region and its organs, it is surely not too much to ask any intelligent person to devote rather less than seven minutes per day to a system which will certainly enable him to look well and feel well, and *be well*. Good health not only adds to the joy of life ; it is a decided asset in the business world, improving one's appearance, and postponing the onset of signs of old age.

In the following pages it will be necessary to take a brief excursion over the somewhat wide field of general principles, but the predominant feature, the keynote of the argument, as the reader will discover, is summed up in the word *posture*. For is not exercise a series of postures ; yea, more, are not thought and speech the preliminary formation of all postures ?

II

SEWAGE SYSTEM OF THE BODY

In an article entitled "The Sewage System of the Human Body," contributed to *American Medicine*, of May, 1923, Sir Arbuthnot Lane advances powerful arguments in support of the theory that the terrible scourge of cancer may be directly the result of neglect of intestinal sanitation. He draws a striking analogy between the sewage system of a town and the gastro-intestinal system of the body. He shows how the blockage of a main sewer has as a direct result far-reaching consequences, disastrous to the dwellers in the area which is drained normally by the sewer.

As houses situated on the higher ground suffer later, and perhaps in different degree, so also the various organs of the body suffer differently in time and kind from the effects of constipation. Constipation being nothing more nor less than interference with the outflow of the individual's sewage, the mere indication of the parallel might

6

almost be considered sufficient. But when it is borne in mind how widespread is this vice of civilisation, and how casual, and almost contented, is the general attitude towards it, the urgency of the subject becomes apparent. If the ordinary man or woman were confronted for the first time with the offensive contents of a constipated large bowel, and were told that the body he or she thinks so much about, decks out in fine raiment, and fears to part from more than he fears anything else in the world, was the casket of such a jewel the shock and disgust might almost prove fatal. Lifelong association with these things has bred the contempt of familiarity, the oblivion to the painfully obvious. Sir Arbuthnot Lane's rapier thrust through this armour of complacent forget-fulness lets a flood of light into the dirty corners of our human dust-bins.

The food which is broken up in the mouth, and subjected to the digestive action of stomach and small intestine, parts with its nutritive principles in a liquid absorbable form as it is moved on-wards until it reaches the large gut, or colon. Here the excess of watery fluid is absorbed and returned to the system, while the refuse, for which we have no use, is slowly passed onwards, to be eventually ejected. During its transit through the stomach and small intestine, few if any micro-organisms are present in the healthy person; but when it passes into the colon it becomes a mass of microbes, which multiply exceedingly. As long as the walls of the gut remain healthy no harm seems to accrue to the individual from this teeming population, but the balance is subject to breakdown from various causes.

It has been demonstrated by the distinguished surgeon, in the above quoted article, that the presence of the large intestine is not essential to the individual; in fact, it can at times "be removed without detriment, and in certain conditions with the greatest benefit."

The liver acts as a filter and refinery for all the fluid absorbed from the intestines, and prepares such materials as pass through it for admittance to the general blood stream. Thus, the tissues of the body are renewed and nourished, the waste products finding their way out by means of the urine, fæces, sweat and breath. In the complex chemical and bacteriological processes occurring in the large intestine many poisonous substances are formed, and the continual absorption of these, as happens in chronic constipation, has very serious results for the individual.

One cannot live over a cesspit in good health. How much more difficult to remain well if we carry our cesspit about inside us—especially

when, as so often happens, the cesspit is un-
pleasantly full !

Even as in civilised communities where cess-
pool "sanitation" so-called is the practice, the
emptying of these horrible receptacles is a work
of infrequent and hurried execution, a work of
darkness and stealth, so also amongst all civilised
peoples the emptying of their individual cesspools
is a matter of shame, to be performed in secret,
and at as long intervals as mechanical requirements permit.

Food is taken several times daily, often too
frequently, and too freely and of unsuitable
quality; but, as a rule, one occasion only is per-
mitted for the ejection of its waste materials.
And remember that all the time this lagging
tenant of the bowel is retained the conditions
favouring evil are at work ; heat, moisture, nitro-
genous refuse, darkness and micro-organisms.
The slow poison factory is in full swing, and its
output is turned into the highways and byeways
of the body.

All the organs and tissues do not react alike
to these malign influences. In some cases the
nervous system bears the brunt of the attack, as
evidenced by headaches, sleeplessness, irritability
of temper, and diminished mental vigour ; in
others, the circulatory system suffers, changes

taking place in the blood vessels of brain, liver, kidneys, and the muscular apparatus, leading to high blood pressure, apoplexy, Bright's disease, rheumatism, jaundice, and muscular weakness; in others again the reproductive functions are deranged, as noticed in many of the disorders of women; while the skin gives to all who care to read the open avowal of a closed outlet for dirt.

Now this chronic poisoning, with its attendant deterioration of body tissue and organs, though not in itself a proved cause of cancer, may, and probably does, predispose to its occurrence when certain structures are the seat of recurring irritation. In parts of the bowel where, owing to anatomical details (the description of which is outside the scope of this book), difficulty is presented to the passage of hard and putrid fæcal matter the conditions are favourable to the growth of cancer, since the irritation is constant, and the membranes unhealthy in consequence. The frequent occurrence of cancer in these situations supports the view taken.

Another source of injury is to be found in the potent purgative drugs employed by persons who suffer from difficult bowel action. It is to be noted that the subjects of cancer of the large intestine are those of muscular and vigorous habit of body. In those persons the bowel shares the

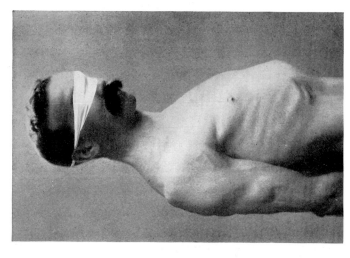

FIG. 2. Shows the same subject with the errors corrected after a course of training by myself. Note the improved musculature and pose.

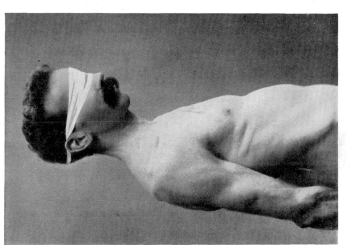

FIG. I. Shows the general external appearance of the body in faulty attitude, with dropped internal organs (Enteroptosis).

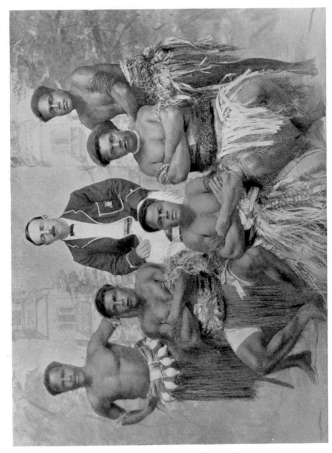

FIG. 3. A group of Fijian pupils of mine whose splendid physique scarcely needs emphasising. The ease of posture in both seated and standing attitudes is well shown.

general muscularity, with the result that by its very over-development the mischief is aggravated; more force is exerted in the propulsion of the hardened matter than would occur in normal cases, additional muscle bands develop and kink the tube, constrictions are accentuated, and much friction and damage are caused at these points by the hard fæcal lumps.

In another class of cases, where general enfeeblement is present, constipation also exists; but here the picture is different. Instead of the strong and muscular gut, with its kinks and narrowings, we have a flaccid dilated tube, incapable of pushing its contents onwards. All the internal organs are inclined to drop downwards and crowd into the pelvis, setting up a state called *enteroptosis*, or dropping of the intestines. The intestine being unable to empty itself, the unfortunate sufferer must have recourse to frequent enemata to remove the stagnant morass which is fermenting in his belly. His digestion is a mockery, gurgling and groaning in hopeless disability, his breath reminiscent of a Limburger cheese, and his general outlook upon life a pessimistic wail. In these people it is rare to see cancer of the bowel, the factor of injury being absent.

That beauty is but skin deep is only half a

truth.   If it draws its nourishment from poisoned sources it must wilt and vanish.   Truly it were better to say that beauty starts from the stomach and ends at the epidermis.   And between these two lie all the potentialities of health and beauty of mind and body.   The external world reflects the mentality of the observer.   Look at it with jaundiced eyes, and it gives back the yellow tinge of misery; smile at it with the clear vision of health, and it invites you into its rose gardens and sunshine.

A negative support of the constipation-cancer theory is furnished in the fact that amongst many of the uncivilised races the disease is unknown. Thus, Sir Arbuthnot Lane reports that Colonel R. McCarrison, I.M.S., "never saw one case of asthenic dyspepsia, of gastric or duodenal ulcer, of appendicitis, or mucous colitis, or of cancer " in the Himalayas, where he did an enormous practice during nine years.   Again, Dr. Hoffman did not see "a single case of cancer" during seven months amongst native Indians and mixed bloods in South America, nor could he hear of one, although he made careful search.

These two instances are not exceptional.   The absence of cancer in uncivilised peoples is a well authenticated fact.   Its rapid increase of late years probably cannot be attributed to a better diagnosis alone. Modern conditions are effecting many changes, and the increasing amount of malignant disease appears to be one. If by an intelligent interpretation and application of natural sanitary principles it is possible to place the individual in a better position to meet an insidious enemy, no small achievement can be claimed. It will be my endeavour to explain how this may be done by a system of physical exercise localised to the abdominal area.

III

In this age of scientific progress it is curious that our ideals concerning man's figure, posture, and gait should be based on the product of the drill sergeant's activities. The Noah's ark figures of the parade ground are not one whit less ridiculous than the fantastic goose-step of the Germans. Contrast the easy bearing, grace of movement, and general muscular activity of any of the native races, such as the Zulus, Polynesians, or Red Indians. I never saw any soldiers walk so easily and so well as the Fijians. They are magnificent men and hold their bodies superbly.

Picture in the mind's eye the position of a soldier standing at attention and the position of any native man, such as a Fijian. In the former the back is "hollowed" and the chest thrust forwards and upwards in the attempt to make the man as like a pouter pigeon as possible. This hollowing of the back naturally forces the abdomen forward, to counteract which the belly muscles are held in a state of tonic contraction, taking their pull from the held-up ribs above and the pelvic brim below. Such a position becomes fatiguing very quickly. The freedom of chest movement being restricted, inspiration is interfered with, and the individual can only maintain his unnatural position by a mental effort, the duration of which depends on circumstances. Even the military martinet has to own a limitation to his authority over men's bodies, and complies with nature's demands by giving

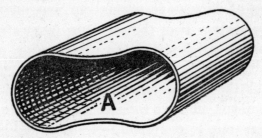

FIG. 6.—This sketch shows diagrammatically the idea conveyed by the text: a section taken through the body at about waist line would resemble the open end of the tube A.

the order to "march easy," when the parade ground is superseded by the open road.

In the Polynesian we see the attitude adopted by man untrammelled by geegaws and trappings of civilisation. Here the shoulders appear to drop downwards and slightly backward ; the ribs are not held up; the back is not hollowed; and the abdomen maintains itself in a somewhat flattened form, almost like the inner tube of a motor-car tyre held up when removed from the tyre and partially deflated. In this position there is complete mobility of the chest; hence respiration is performed unconsciously and perfectly. The freedom of head, neck and shoulder movements allowed by the easy position of the chest contributes largely to alertness and comfort, and reduces fatigue to a minimum. As the abdomen shares the responsibility of the respiratory phenomena to a considerable extent, it is obvious that its condition has direct relation to the chest. Thus the contained organs stand in correct relation to each other and to their containing walls. There is neither sagging nor protruberance, therefore the functions of digestion will be performed with the same physiological ease as those of respiration. And when we remember how dependent on the efficient performance of these processes are the other functions of the body, we see the imperative necessity of placing them under the best possible conditions.

Consider now the posture usually adopted by the town dweller, the man of sedentary habits, whose business has little or nothing to do with the welfare of his body. Here it will be noticed that the head is carried in the peering position; chest contracted by the forward drop of the shoulders and depression of the breast-bone;

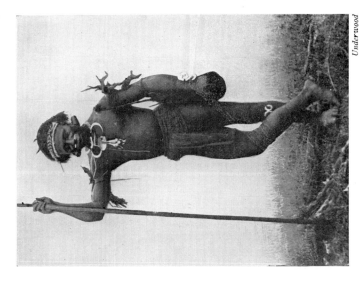

Underwood

FIG. 5. Note the ease of attitude of the Polynesian native warrior shown here.

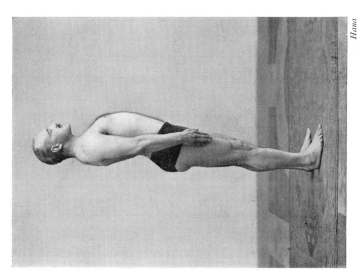

Hana

FIG. 4. The military position at attention. Note the pouter pigeon chest and hollow back.

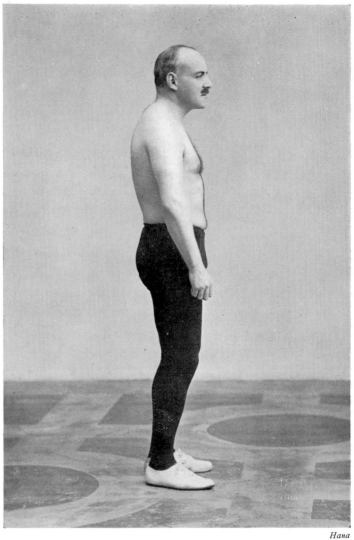

FIG. 7. The faulty attitude usually adopted by civilised man.

the lumbar spine bent in the opposite direction to that known as "hollow"; and the belly lax and more or less protruberant. This is the natural consequence of habit and environment, fatigue and pre-occupation; and is largely responsible for many of the physical troubles which begin to crowd upon the man of early middle life.

There is a well-known aphorism—more apt than elegant—which says that "after forty men put on weight in front, and women behind." This is so universal that it is regarded as inevitable; but it frequently is the corollary of life habits of eating and drinking and neglect of exercise. Our conception of physical beauty is the result of Greek influence. In all that has come down to us through the ages from ancient Greece, we have not one solitary instance of a beautiful form fashioned in fatness. The modern tailor and modiste may tax their ingenuity to the breaking point, but the greatest of these cannot hide the protruberant belly or the ponderous buttocks which handicap fat people in their cumbrous waddle through life. It is true that "by taking thought a man cannot add a cubit to his stature," but it is equally true that by taking suitable exercise and obeying the elementary laws of hygiene a man (or woman) can subtract a good deal of material from his total weight. And in doing it he will add to his general well-being.

This illustration again depicts the effect of an undue development of fat in and about the abdomen, and is by strange perversion of taste usually considered the natural culmination of man's physical excellence. Falstaff and Bluff King Hal were better in legend than in one's own person. The happy medium between these and "the lean and slippered pantaloon" is the desideratum to strive after, and in most cases the attainment is not impossible.

To carry the undue load, the shoulders have to be thrown backwards, and the head carried somewhat stiffly and further back than normal, while the lumbar spine is hollowed. This adaptation to need is seen in exactly the same way in the pregnant woman. The position is somewhat similar to that of the soldier on parade, but with certain differences. In the soldier the heavy abdominal mass is absent, but the hollowing of the back exists; the shoulders are pulled directly backwards without any of the downward tendency observable in the man of weight, so that the chest may be thrust as far forward as possible, while the head is held stiffly in both. In the soldier the abdomen is held rigidly, owing to the pull of the abdominal muscles, as already explained, which are stretched by the elevated ribs, and its capacity is further diminished by the thrusting forward of the lumbar spine.

The alignment of the spinal column for the correct posture in standing is without undue curve of the lumbar portion. If the reader, standing up well but not too stiffly, will gently push in his abdomen with both hands, he will find that he has not *hollowed* his back, but simply straightened his spine to some extent. Whenever the abdomen is retracted, the lower part of the spine is *not* hollowed, but rather straightened. Five minutes practical observation opposite a mirror will convince the most sceptical on this point.

Precisely the same principles apply in regard to man's posture when seated. The correct sitting posture is to use the same living belt of muscle and prevent the sagging forward of the abdomen and its contents. The way to attain this result is *not* to sit in a stiff awkward position with the chest thrust out, but rather to press the buttocks well against the lower part of the chair-back. This is a much more comfortable and easy position than is generally realised.

The greatest benefit results from correct

posture when sitting at the meal table. Illustration No. 11 (*see* opposite p. 50) shows the wrong posture adopted by most men and women. Here the buttocks are some distance from the chair-back, and thus unsupported ; the breast-bone is depressed ; the abdomen protruding and relaxed ; and often the knees are drawn up and the weight rests on the toes.

The mechanical phenomena occurring in the body in this wrong posture are as follows :—

Owing to the depression of the breast-bone and general relaxation of the chest walls, the diaphragm is lower ; as a result the stomach and all the digestive organs become somewhat crowded, and perhaps slightly displaced downwards. Some interference with blood supply and bowel movement is almost inevitable. Consequently the process of digestion is retarded, and by constant repetition becomes impaired.

The body and the mind work in unison, and what affects the body deleteriously naturally affects the mind in a similar way. The mental depression and irritability of temper seen in liver attacks illustrate this. On the other hand, when the correct posture is adopted, as in Fig. 12 (*see* opposite p. 50), and good digestion waits on good appetite, a man rises from the table refreshed in mind as well as in body.

As indicated above, correctness of posture and freedom from artificial restrictions are of even greater importance when the body is making effort, calling for increased respiratory action and tissue change; therefore the need of correct posture during walking—the most usual, with some the only, form of exercise habitual amongst us. I have shown how the soldier when on the march must discard the gait of the strutting pigeon, and walk after the manner mother nature first instructed him in. The unbooted savage does not turn out his toes, as does civilised man; neither does he turn his toes inwards. It is not possible for the ordinary man or woman to walk as the savage does, because our feet have become distorted by boots, and our freedom of action is impaired by clothing and habit. But that there is great room for improvement goes without saying. This habit of correct posture should be maintained *even when walking quickly*, but naturally the length of the stride is increased.

IV

ENTEROPTOSIS AND THINNESS

In connection with these conditions, it may be well to point out that the state known to medical men as *enteroptosis* is not by any means present in all cases of thinness, or that it is confined to thin people alone. When it occurs it gives rise to a well-marked group of symptoms, which eventually drives the sufferer to seek the aid of a medical man. Generally speaking, the treatment may be said to consist of the adoption of some form of abdominal belt, since it is almost impossible to restore the stretched and displaced abdominal contents to their original position. The employment of suitable exercises helps to restore general muscle tone; thereby the abdominal regions receive much assistance. Corsets, so often the refuge of women weak in body, do not help in the slightest degree, since by their splint-like effect the mischief is increased as the muscles are more or less put out of use. The only way to keep muscle fit is to exercise it.

Women who suffer from weakened abdominal muscles feel "all-gone" when they discard their corsets. An abdominal belt, such as that made by Messrs. H. Curtis & Son, of 7, Mandeville Place, London, W. 1, appears to meet the requirements. It need hardly be said that each case has to be fitted individually. In such an apparatus the support is distributed from before backwards, in such a manner that the sides of the abdomen are practically free from any pressure, the groins and lower abdomen alone being supported. Thus, the muscular walls of the abdomen are given opportunity to develop and enabled to sustain the contained organs.

There are many thin people of both sexes who do not suffer from any muscular weakness, and whose general health appears excellent. Such people naturally do not require or seek assistance. Others again, who though neither the subjects of any wasting disease or any coarse physical defect, such as enteroptosis, are constantly below par. They may eat well—too well, perhaps—yet they never appear well nourished. This may in part be due to faulty assimilation of food, and in part to sedentary habits, hurried meals, and mental worry. A constitutional tendency to spareness of body is not to be overlooked.

Where digestive errors exist they should be corrected, and as a rule the response to treatment in this class of case is prompt. Suitable exercises improve the digestion by increasing the peristaltic action of the bowel. If it be borne in mind that the intestines are muscular tubes, and, further, that muscular tissue responds to the stimulus of massage or kneading, then the good effects of a sound abdominal wall are explained by its action in kneading and pressing the contained organs. As the intestinal muscles are thus wakened into activity, they ensure the propulsion of the bowel contents, and stagnation is prevented.

Food may be likened to fuel in a steam engine. If the furnace be packed with coal beyond its efficient working capacity the head of steam drops. In like manner unskilful stoking, or unsuitable food, brings about the same result. Too much food, food badly packed inside, or food of a deficient nutritive quality, produces loss of vigour and malnutrition.

V

FLAT FEET

The normal healthy foot! How many people have ever noticed that a footprint on the hard sand, or the imprint of a wet foot on the floor, shows not the outline of the whole sole, but instead a disjointed pattern, produced by the heel, the outer line of the sole, the points where the ball of foot rested, and the rounded dabs left by the ends of the toes?

This appearance is due to the arched shape of the foot, one large arch extending from the ball of the foot to the heel, and a short one extending across the front, behind the base of the toes. This arched arrangement is maintained by powerful ligamentous structures in the sole of the foot, and when from any cause they lose their function, becoming over-stretched, the arches are said to "drop." The foot then rests on the ground for its whole length. The results of this are that the gait becomes shuffling, the spring being lost. Pain and fatigue accompany the distortion as the bones of the foot are pressed on the ground, and in addition to limitation of function, grace of movement is destroyed, while headache, backache, and general weariness help to complete the misery of the subject.   Persons who become fat and too heavy for their plantar arches become flat-footed. Others again who, through ill-health, lose tone of tissue, or those whose avocations in life entail much standing, such as policemen, nurses, shop assistants, waiters, etc., are all subject to the condition.   How widespread is the evil is manifested by the large number of advertisements one sees daily extolling the different "supports." In his book "Exercise in Education and Medicine," page 240, Dr. R. Tait McKenzie says : "In an examination of a thousand supposedly normal students I have found it (flat-foot) in two hundred and seventeen cases."

Once the condition of flat-foot becomes established, cure in the sense of restoration of the pristine state is out of the question.   But much may be done to improve the sufferer's disability by suitable exercises, and in cases where the body-weight is excessive this may be considerably reduced with marked benefit.   Dancing and walking on tip-toe, combined with Exercise V, will materially help to improve the muscle tone and have a marked effect on the feet.   At times it may be necessary to practise a complete system of suitable foot exercises, combined with massage, for a long period before betterment is achieved; and it is seldom that a case occurs which proves wholly unamenable to treatment. All cases of flat-foot require suitable boots. Shoes are not to be recommended.

The best form of boot is one which allows a certain amount of freedom to the toes, while giving the necessary support. The inner line of the boot-sole from toe to heel should be in a straight line, the inner side of the sole and heel should be a little thicker than the outer, and the " waist " of the boot should fit well and be fairly stiff.

VI

EXERCISE AFTER OPERATION

In those who have recently undergone an *abdominal* operation there is a natural tendency to walk with care, avoiding anything in the nature of free striding. This somewhat stiff and timid gait is the subconscious effort to prevent strain or jar. This practice, if persisted in, as it is apt to be in persons of advancing years, becomes habitual, and may conduce through the faulty gait and loss of muscle tone to the development of some degree of flat-foot. The remedy is to strengthen the abdominal walls, and thereby get rid of the feeling of insecurity present in these cases. By this means the tenderness that occasionally lingers about the wound gradually disappears and confidence is ultimately restored.

In massage we have a powerful aid for the restoring of muscle tissue which has suffered through disuse, and its early and judicious employment after operations is now a recognised measure all over the civilised world. The appli-

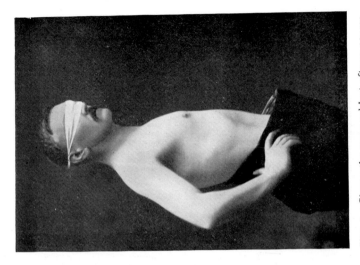

FIG. 9. Shows the same subject after a course of treatment by me. Note the striking change in general contour and condition.

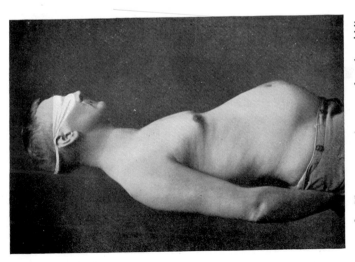

FIG. 8. Here we see the man of early middle life whose abdomen has become pendulous and protuberant, due to excessive local fat deposit and faulty posture.

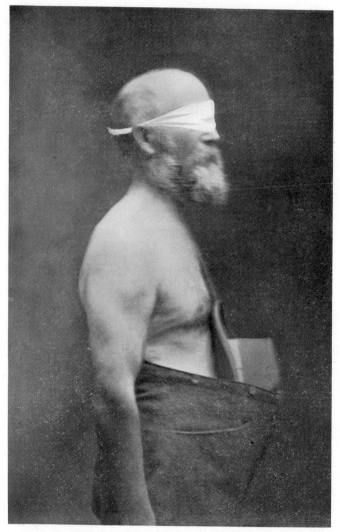

FIG. 10. Depicts an older subject where the decrease in girth after
my treatment is indicated by the loose waist belt. This man
was 65 years of age.

cation of massage should be no haphazard
rubbing; to obtain its full benefits it must be
carried out by a skilled operator who combines
suitable passive, and, at times, graduated active
movements with the rubbing, kneading and other
manipulative processes grouped under the general
term "massage."

After pregnancy, again, we see a state of muscle
flabbiness, especially in the stretched abdominal
muscles. Until recently the only means adopted
to "restore the figure" was the application of a
tight abdominal binder. It certainly gives the
patient a feeling of comfort by the support
afforded, but, so far as helping to restore the
muscles to their normal state, the binder might
as well have been tied round the bedstead.
Much good follows the employment of massage,
and early muscle movements, in these cases. If
such routine became universal one would hear
less often the complaint that the after-treatment
had been careless, and that the patient's figure
had not been restored to its normal dimensions.
I urge every woman, unless there be some definite
contra-indication, to have recourse to skilled
massage after the birth of her child, and I can
promise her that the result will justify the means.

When the patient enters upon the "walking
about stage" after abdominal operations, such as

VII

FAULTS OF THE USUAL SYSTEMS OF EXERCISE

THE following are the chief defects in the usual systems of physical training:—

1. The time occupied per day is usually too long for the average man to devote to what he is apt to consider an uninteresting task.
2. The systems involve a very large number of movements, many of which affect only the arms and legs.
3. Those affecting the internal abdominal organs are always done with the abdominal walls rigid, which has the effect of squeezing and fixing the internal organs, thus preventing the free action of the involuntary muscles of the intestines.
4. A few minutes exercise per day is not sufficient to counteract wrong posture habitually adopted.
5. Practically in all standing movements the stiff military position is adopted.

6. The muscles of the waist-line are largely neglected, while those of the limbs are subjected to relatively excessive action.

7. In breathing exercises, instead of standing with the ribs mobile and expanding the chest as the lungs are filled, the chest is forced forwards and *afterwards* the lungs are filled. This method causes chest rigidity (a spirometer reading will show that the vital capacity is less when this procedure is adopted than in the former case).

8. Too often the cultivation of muscle for the mere sake of muscle is the be-all and end-all of the training.

9. Failure of recognition of the particular object to be attained.

VIII

GOLF AS EXERCISE

To approach golf in any but a spirit of enthusiasm is to confess oneself heretic or madman. Its place is more assured than the philosophy of Confucius. Therefore I hasten to make public avowal of my orthodoxy. It calls the man from the city, the maid from the mill, it lures the matron from the cares of her nursery and the bookworm from his arm-chair. The politician and the parson meet the soldier and the son of Neptune on the shorn green; and all derive some measure of good, some touch of pleasure, some breath of freedom on the windy downs. But— and there is always a "but" in things !—golf is not quite sinless. The man who plays strenuous golf once or twice a week while the remainder of the time is spent in close application to business does not well. While youth is with him, impunity holds his hand, and as the years drag behind, and as the abdomen drops before, he is asking his heart to do more work than nature meant it for.

34

No doubt he grows hungry in the fresh air, and the desire is frequently not limited to solid nourishment alone, but inclines to alcohol. Carrying a somewhat weighty abdomen around the countryside one or two days a week will not help in any way to improve his condition or lessen his burden. That general exercise does *not* reduce weight to any extent is a fact well known to physicians. Speaking of particular exercises, such as fencing, Dr. Harry Campbell, in his admirable book, "Respiratory Exercises" (1898), says :—

> "It may be observed in passing that all muscle exercises do not cause fat to disappear at the same rate all over the body. The fat tends to be absorbed chiefly in the neighbourhood of the muscles most actively employed. Thus, if a stout man takes to fencing, the loss of fat takes place chiefly about the chest. And similarly rope-hauling, which calls the abdominal muscles into active play, is especially calculated to remove fat from the belly."

These sentences, with golf as a text, might be written with equal verity. Let the golfer of middle age, whose waist-line is not what it was in the years gone by, take up a system of abdominal control exercises, and put the principles I advocate into practice, he will soon become a disciple of girth control, his diminishing waist measurement being the inverse measure of his increasing fitness, his improved bodily condition being reflected in his brighter mental outlook, while his capacity for work keeps pace with his inclination for play.

Here a word of warning may not be out of place. Up to the end of August, 1923, the death roll placed to the discredit of golf totalled eleven. An eminent London doctor is quoted in the press as having expressed the opinion that fifty is the " danger age " for golfers. He pointed out that swinging is the most strenuous part of golf, and may be dangerous after the arteries have become rigid.

Men are loth to admit the onset of age, and are often blind to the sign-posts which border the pathway. The aphorism that "a man is as old as his arteries" is as widely known as it is universally disregarded. When we are suddenly faced with disaster as it overtakes men whose blood vessels give way, we are perhaps prone to call a momentary halt. But inclination, fostering forgetfulness, we take up the running again, ignoring the possibility of ourselves being the individual who may provide the material for the next newspaper paragraph.

Golf, I repeat, is not so sinless as its votaries would claim ; but, on the other hand, it must not have laid at its door the consequences of disregarded dictates of common sense and ordinary prudence.

The indulgence in golf, as in all other forms of exercise, ought to be gauged by the fitness of the player; and how many seek a skilled medical opinion before taking up the pastime, or continuing in it after they have arrived at the " danger age?"

As pointed out elsewhere, the adoption of the correct posture very soon becomes quite unconscious, on the golf links as elsewhere. No mental effort is required, the attention is not diverted from the game itself; rather the player finds himself not only able to play a more enjoyable game, but a much better game, and with far less fatigue.

D

IX

APPLICATION OF SYSTEM OF ABDOMINAL CONTROL

THE question has now to be considered : To whom does this system apply? It applies particularly to the following :—

1. To business men whose time is so fully occupied that they must, of necessity, have some system of exercise of a "tabloid" nature.
2. To all those men and women who suffer from constipation.
3. To delicate people trying to build up their strength by dietetic measures alone—and often trying unsuccessfully.
4. To all those who suffer from digestive troubles of any kind.
5. To athletes, many of whom, despite the great amount of general exercise they take, suffer from digestive disorders, because they have built up muscular strength while neglecting their abdominal hygiene.

6. To ex-athletes, who in middle age tend to become loaded with layers of fat, particularly round and in the abdominal region (notice the ex-athletes acting as officials at any sports meetings, boxing contests, etc.).

This voluntary contraction can be practised quietly without in any way attracting attention. It need not be done so often that it becomes tiresome—just at odd times during the day in disengaged moments ; for remember, it can be carried out invisibly, and (as I said before) in any position.

Lying along the whole length of the spinal column, on its frontal aspect, is a curious complicated system of nervous structures called "the sympathetic system." It consists of bundles of nerves, which in places appear to unite and swell into little lumps like knots in string. One of these groups of knots is placed on the first lumbar vertebra and behind the stomach. It is known as "the solar plexus." Its interest for us lies in the fact that a blow received on the abdominal wall over this region may have grave or even fatal consequences for a person whose muscular development is feeble. This effect is well known to pugilists. The result of a blow delivered over this area is a general collapse, varying in degree on the measure of violence and the muscular development and preparedness of the person struck. This sympathetic nervous apparatus is intimately associated with the function of the abdominal organs, and is sometimes spoken of as "the abdominal brain." That a good muscular tone will not only protect it from injury, but may also conduce to a better discharge of its functions, is highly probable; hence the importance of securing and maintaining this condition.

be recommended. Taken before breakfast and between meals, in liberal quantities, hot or cold, it is extremely beneficial. In a newspaper article published recently, Sir H. E. Bruce Bruce-Porter, K.B.E., C.M.G., M.D., etc., states :—

"The value of water to the outer world is immense. But to man it is the main factor of his existence. Without it life would be impossible. Two-thirds of the body-weight is water ; more than that in bulk. The minimum quantity of water, taken as such, should be three pints a day; and an occasional day on short rations of food, with an increase in water drinking, would bring as its reward a sense of well-being. If you are called an hour before breakfast, and during that hour drink a pint of water slowly while doing a few exercises and while dressing, it washes out waste material which is rapidly secreted by the kidneys and carried away; another tumblerful an hour before mid-day and another before the evening."

As a rule, the appetite and taste must be allowed to regulate the individual's diet, both as to the quantity and kind of food taken. But proper habits of eating should be cultivated. There is no doubt that most sedentary workers eat too much, and hence put on fat as a direct result. Fat is a severe punishment for excess in diet, and though of course excessive weight can be reduced by exercise, no system of exercise should be considered as giving a mandate for over-eating. What is taken off by exercise is put on again by gluttony. Moderation here, as elsewhere, is the golden rule.

And health depends on the proper correlation of all the factors.

The cumulative effects of worry must also be considered, in so far as they tend to derange digestion. Generally speaking, the results of constant worry may be seen in liver derangement, sluggish bowel action, with much flatulence, nervous irritability, sleeplessness, and increased blood pressure. For men over forty this is almost axiomatic. Women suffer from worry effects more in other ways, but increased blood pressure is not unknown among them. These serious consequences are of slow development, but it must be borne in mind that there are also immediate effects at the time of ingestion of food.

Thus, a man who swallows his meal while in a state of mental pre-occupation, or while experiencing the emotions of anger or excitement, is not in a condition to deal satisfactorily with the food which he puts into his stomach. It is well known that people taking their meals under these conditions suffer from acute indigestion. A mind at rest is as essential for the digestive process as a stomach in activity. For the due performance of its functions it is necessary that the stomach be supplied with an additional quantity of blood. While the mind is actively engaged, or the emotions aroused, the brain makes a call upon the circulation, with the consequence that the stomach suffers loss of blood when most requiring it. The habitual repetition of this state of affairs produces a chronic impairment of the digestion.

In conclusion, some people may say that all this is too much trouble, and that they have not time to consider their health. Such people do not think it too much trouble to carry round a distended and overloaded gut. People who say they have not time to take paraffin and hot water usually find time to get constipation. As a rule, the time they *waste* in the lavatory is more than sufficient to drink all the water and paraffin necessary.

For the neglect of our bodies, for over-indulgence, for laziness, we have all to pay the price one way or another, and that price is usually a heavy one. On the other hand, for a small expenditure of time and trouble we gain efficiency of body, alertness of mind, and a general feeling of well-being.

PART TWO

RULES OF EXERCISE

It is not possible to formulate any arbitrary set of rules applicable to every case alike. It is obvious that each individual must be guided by such conditions as environment, occupation, age, sex, muscular development, general health, and any peculiar personal factors which may exist. Some general principles are common to all, such as the following :—

1. Exercise should not be taken for some time (say one and a half to two hours) after a meal, as the stomach then demands a greater share of blood, and if by voluntary effort this is deflected to the muscles the digestion suffers.

2. Exercise before having your bath. Whether the bath is hot or cold depends on the individual. Cold baths are unsuitable for many people.

3. The clothing worn during exercise should be warm and loose. For men—sweater, pants, and slippers ; for women—golf jersey, bloomers, shoes and stockings (no corsets.

4. Fresh air, always a necessity, is doubly necessary during exercise. Keep the windows open but avoid draughts.

5. If possible, exercise in front of a mirror—in summer-time exercise stripped to the waist, in order to observe the muscular action controlling the abdominal walls.

6. Persons suffering from obstinate constipation should exercise twice a day for first six weeks; after that once a day may be sufficient.

7. Do not exercise when fatigued. Take a short rest, and then exercise.

N.B.—Don't hold the breath when exercising. Breathe in and out quietly and deeply.

The best time for exercise is immediately on rising. But if this is not convenient, exercise at bed-time.

———

Regular Weighing : A small portable weighing scale should be in the bath-room of every well-ordered house. These can be obtained nowadays for about £2 10s. to £3. If once a week the weight is taken correctly, immediately after the morning bath, and noted down, errors in diet or laxity in exercise, leading to putting on of superfluous fat, or undesirable loss of weight, can be rectified.

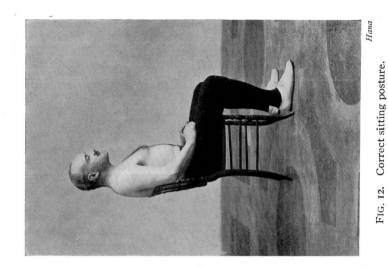

Hana

FIG. 12.   Correct sitting posture.

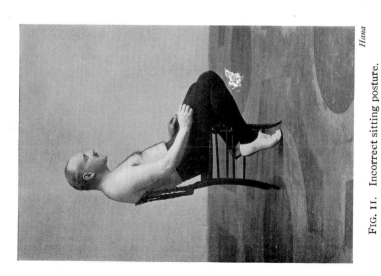

Hana

FIG. 11.   Incorrect sitting posture.

(See p. 20)

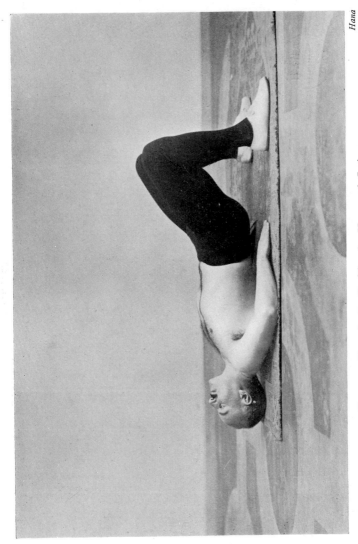

FIG. 13. Exercise I. Position for Hammock Swing.

SYSTEMS OF EXERCISE

I. Hammock Swing

Place a folded blanket on floor. Lie flat on back on the blanket. Bend both knees, soles of feet on the floor; feet about 12 in. apart, and heels close to buttocks. It is advisable for a stout person and for elderly people to put a pillow under the head (*not under shoulders*) to prevent rush of blood to head. Place both hands *flat on floor*. Now raise the hips from floor about 2 in. or 3 in. The body-weight will then rest on the head, shoulders and feet. Vigorously swing the body from side to side, keeping the shoulders flat on the floor, so as to throw each hip upwards alternately.

Repeat 20 times—10 each side. Lower hips to floor. Rest for five seconds.

This constitutes one complete cycle.

Raise again, and continue six cycles of 20 beats each; that is, 120 swings with six rests.

This exercise from beginning to end will take about 1½ minutes in all. At first it is best to make each of the cycles consist of six beats, and gradually work up to 20 beats to each movement. With practice the beats will naturally be done more rapidly.

Don't hold the breath.

Rest between each cycle.

The great advantage of this exercise is that, the abdomen being held loosely, the movement raise only the head and not the shoulders, and keep feet on floor, or raise the feet only a few inches. At the end of a week raise head and feet a little higher, and so on, avoiding strain, until complete contraction is obtained.

It is better to inhale on the upward movement and exhale on the downward movement, then retract abdomen, contracting buttocks. Pause for a second or two. Then inhale and repeat movement.

Don't hold the breath.

Don't do this exercise as a breathing exercise.

At the end of a few weeks, when feeling stronger, the following movement may be added: Raise shoulders and legs as above, pause for a second, then try and raise shoulders and legs still further ; lower, and complete the movement.

The action of the abdominal wall is something like the opening and shutting of a concertina.

Begin by doing this movement six times, gradually increasing up to eighteen times.

NOTE.—In cases of hernia (rupture), it is necessary that the truss or support should always be worn when doing this and all other exercises.

For the elderly and the stout person, the use of a pillow under the head is advisable in Exercises I, II and III.

IV

LATERAL PRESS

THIS exercise is for the oblique and transversalis abdominal muscles—two very important muscles which compress the viscera and flex the thorax. It is most beneficial to the liver, alternately squeezing and releasing this organ.

Stand with feet some 6 in. apart, toes turned out slightly. Place hands on hips, thumbs back. Bend slightly forward from the shoulders—not from the hips. Now try and retract the lower abdomen, and, holding it retracted, lean well over to the left side, contracting the muscles of the left side forcibly, but keeping chest muscles loose. Keep legs straight all the time—knees stiff. Reverse to right side. Repeat 20 times—10 right, 10 left.

This exercise is done slowly and steadily without jerking. Breathe quietly and deeply, in and out through the nostrils.

Don't hold the breath.

Three or four movements from side to side can be done on the inhalation, and three or four on the exhalation, after a little practice.

This exercise may seem familiar to some readers, but it is safe to say that in ninety per cent. of cases it is done incorrectly. Sir Arthur Keith, in his Hunterian Lecture * on " Man's Posture," speaking of the transversalis muscle, says :—

> "The supporting structures are the muscles of the belly wall ; particularly is the transversalis muscle important in this respect ; it is a living belt which girds the loins."

* *British Medical Journal*, April 7th, 1923, page 558.

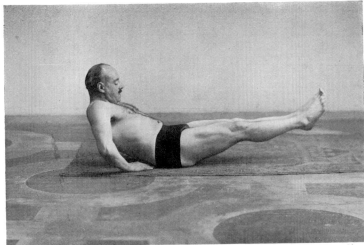

Hana

FIG. 14. Exercise II. Tensing.

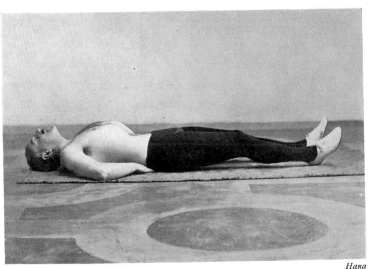

Hana

FIG. 15. Exercise II. Retracting.

Facing p. 54

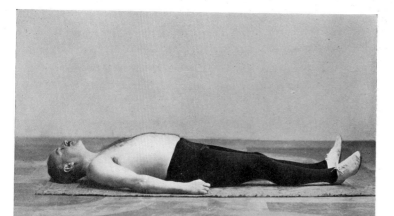

FIG. 16. Exercise III. Pumping, 1st position. *Hana*

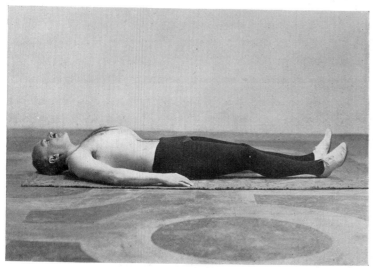

FIG. 17. Exercise III. Pumping, 2nd position. *Hana*

III

PUMPING

LIE flat on back with muscles relaxed; by muscula effort, push forward the abdominal wall (this accomplished by contraction of the diaphragm then by vigorous converse movement draw the belly. It will be noted that this exercise not dependent upon excessive chest action at During its execution no special breathing rhythm necessary. Assist the movement of the abdo with the hands if necessary. Keep the shoul and hips firmly on the floor. There should b heaving or movement of the shoulders; no fo of the ribs; this is purely a diaphragmatic mover

Don't hold the breath.

Don't do this exercise as a breathing exercise.

At first it is better to inhale slightly abdomen goes forward, and exhale as the ab is pulled in. After a little practice several can be performed on the one breath.

The main object of this movement is to i the peristaltic action of the bowels. Like Ex it can be done by the most delicate wo well as by the strongest athlete. As the tone up the force with which the movemen is increased. This exercise gives a large a internal massage with a comparatively sma of muscular effort.

Repeat twelve times; pause; then repe twelve times slightly quicker.

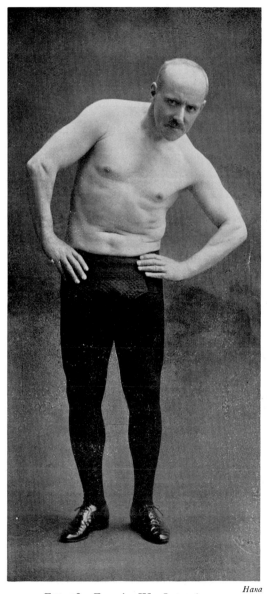

Hana

FIG. 18.   Exercise IV.   Lateral press.

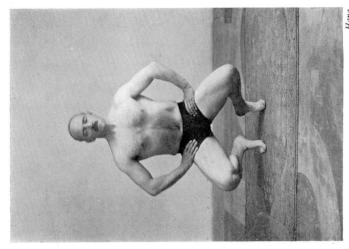

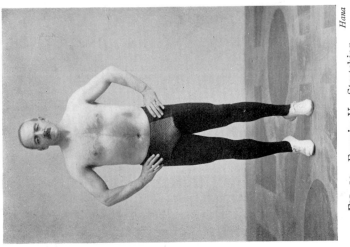

FIG. 20. Exercise V. Squatting.

Hana

FIG. 19. Exercise V. Stretching.

Hana

Facing p. 57

V

STRETCHING AND SQUATTING

Stand with heels fairly close together, toes pointed well out; shoulders braced back and down; abdomen held well in. Hands on hips—thumbs back. Rise on toes; then bending knees outwards, slowly sink to a squatting position, keeping the spine straight, until back of thighs touch the calves of the legs. Then rise slowly to first position, stiffening the knees, and bracing muscles of the thighs. Pause for a second, and with knees still held stiffly, try to rise still further on the toes, stretching the muscles of the calves, and working the ankle joint fully. Repeat from six to twelve times.

At the beginning it is possible some little difficulty may be found in maintaining the balance. If so, hold on to the end of bed, or back of chair, with the hands, instead of placing them on the hips.

In some cases it may be desirable to modify the exercise—say for very stout or delicate persons.

Thus: Hold on to end of bed or back of chair; keeping knees stiff, rise as high as possible on the toes; still keeping knees stiff, lower heels almost to the floor, but don't rest the heels on the floor; that is, the body is supported on the balls of the feet. Repeat until muscles of calf and sole of foot begin to ache slightly. At the end of a few weeks, the full squatting movement should be done. At first, do only a few movements—say, four or five. Increase to twelve movements.

In the exercise itself, and in its modified form, the spine is held straight, the abdomen retracted, and the weight of body thrown slightly backwards. This ensures more work being done by the ankles and the muscles of the feet than would be the case if the weight were thrown forward.   Done properly, this exercise is useful in the prevention of flat-foot.

The breathing in this exercise should be done as follows :—

Exhale on downward and inhale on upward movement.

VI

RETRACTION AND RECOIL

KNEEL on a small pillow or mat, and place both hands on floor, fingers spread as in Fig. 21. Now, while breathing quietly, retract the abdomen fully, at the same time hollowing the back. By a further muscular effort, bring the breast bone nearer the pelvis, squeezing in the abdomen to the greatest possible extent; elbows stiff and head kept steady. This latter part of the exercise is brought about by arching the spine as a cat does when it stretches itself, with the abdomen tucked in, as in Fig. 22.

This completes the movement, which has to be repeated slowly at first, keeping the whole of the muscular apparatus in a state of tension. As facility is acquired, the rapidity of movement can be slightly increased.

If this exercise is done in front of a mirror, so that the contour of the back is visible when the head is turned towards the mirror, it will be seen that a continuous undulatory movement passes up and down the spine, as the spine is alternately arched and hollowed.

This is a full extension and contraction movement.

This exercise brings into play all the muscles of the abdomen.   It has a very beneficial effect in imparting pliability to the spine.

In this exercise *inhale as the back is hollowed, exhale as the back is arched*.   Inhale through nostrils, exhale through mouth.

Begin by doing this movement six times, gradually increasing up to eighteen times.

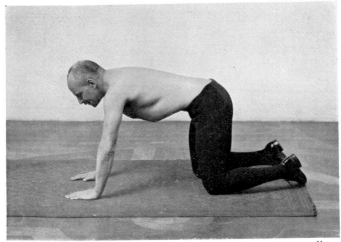

Hana

FIG. 21.   Exercise VI.   Retraction.

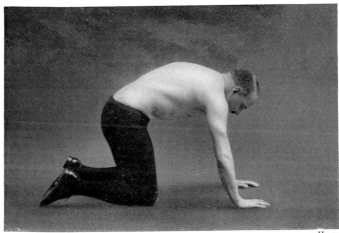

Hana

FIG. 22.   Exercise VI.   Recoil.

Facing p. 60

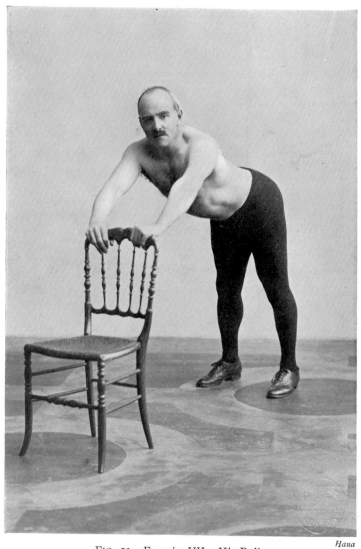

FIG. 23. Exercise VII. Hip Roll.

VII

HIP ROLL

STAND about 3 ft. from low chair, chin up, feet about 12 in. apart, knees straight, abdomen well drawn in. Place hands on back of chair, thumbs back ; grasp chair firmly. Now swing hips to the left, forcing left hip well out. Reverse to right and continue movement. Try and keep knees stationary, or as near to being stationary as possible. Get the swing from the hips with contracted abdomen, but don't let the legs follow the line of the hip roll. This exercise should be performed from the hips as much as possible, with the legs as a steady base, the muscles of the buttocks aiding in the swing from side to side.

A similar hip roll movement is performed by nearly all the natives of Polynesia—Maoris, Fijians, Samoans, etc.—in their body dances. I have seen these performed well on the stage in France and Germany, but I have never seen any white people do them so vigorously as the natives. The movement is not particularly elegant ; neither is a loose and pendulous abdomen. This exercise is certainly effective, not only in promoting abdominal activity, but also in reducing loose sagging tissue, increasing the mobility of the vertebræ, and improving the tone of the muscles of the lumbar region.

In this exercise, breathe quietly and deeply, in and out through the nostrils.   *Don't hold the breath.*

Repeat the movement for some 30 or 40 seconds, at first very slowly, increasing the speed as proficiency is attained.

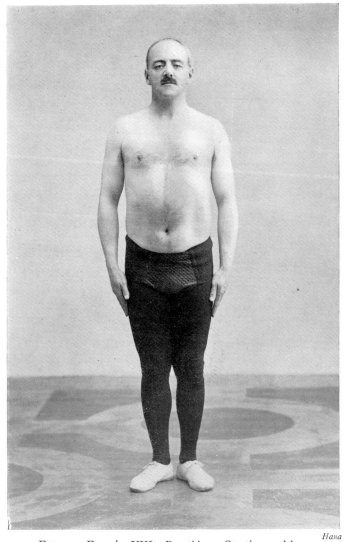

Hana

FIG. 24.   Exercise VIII.   Breathing.   Starting position.

Facing p. 62

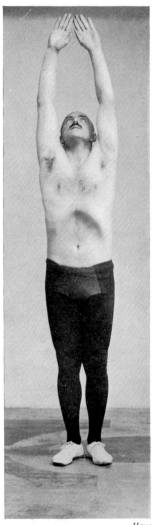

FIG. 25. Exercise VIII. Completion of Inspiration.

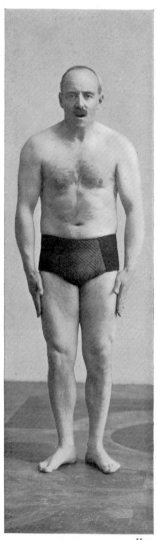

FIG. 26. Exercise VIII. Completion of Respiration.

Facing p. 63

VIII

BREATHING EXERCISE

STAND erect and easily, heels fairly close together, arms by sides, palms inwards. Make a full slow inspiratory effort, commencing and ending with the movement of the arms, as follows :—

Carry the arms outwards from the sides, keeping the palms in the same position, until level of shoulders is reached; continue the movement of the arms upwards, and at the same time turn the palms inwards, so that they meet overhead. The elbows are kept stiff during the whole of this movement. To complete the movement, now turn the palms outwards and bring the arms down slowly and steadily to original position by sides, exhaling during the downward movement. Complete the expiration at the end of this movement by a general voluntary contraction of all the muscles of expiration, so as to empty the lungs as completely as possible.

Inspiration is effected through the nostrils with the mouth closed, while expiration takes place through the open mouth. When inhaling, endeavour to expand the chest from below upwards, that is to say, avoid the error of lifting up or blowing out the upper part of the chest as in military position shown in Fig. 4 (see opposite p. 16).

Repeat six to nine times.

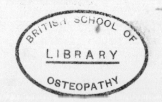

The Author will be pleased to reply personally to any questions regarding the System of Exercise described in this book, if any reader sends a stamped and addressed envelope. The Publishers will forward such letters if sent to their care.

PRINTED BY WOODS AND SONS, LTD., LONDON, N.1.

Physical Fitness in Middle Life

by

F. A. HORNIBROOK

WITH A FOREWORD BY

LEONARD WILLIAMS, M.D.

HIGH MEDICAL TESTIMONY

Sir W. ARBUTHNOT LANE, Bart., C.B., M.S., F.R.C.S.
> "It seems to me that the author has got to the root of the matter in regard to personal and national health—namely, the permanent cultivation of the body."

Dr. BARBARA CRAWFORD.
> "As the latest and freshest exponent of the gospel of physical fitness through self-control, the author is doing invaluable work along original lines."

Sir BRUCE BRUCE-PORTER, K.B.E., C.M.G., M.D.
> "I think the subject matter is very sound, and there are a great many very practical hints which should be most useful."

WHAT THE PRESS SAYS :

"A sensible book, giving plain advice to middle-aged men and women, especially men who feel that they are losing their vigour while still they are not old."—*The Spectator.*

"Mr. F. A. Hornibrook has condensed a great deal of valuable advice on health into his book."—*Birmingham Gazette.*

"Practical advice for busy men who are in danger of becoming unfit at a very critical stage in their lives."—*The Scotsman.*

With Four Half-tone plates, 6s. net

Cassell & Co., Ltd.,   La Belle Sauvage, E.C. 4